Fabian Society No. 529

Life begins at 40: in defence of the NHS

Robin Cook

Fabian Tract 529

Life begins at 40: in defence of the NHS

"A striking personal endorsement of the NHS was provided in 1984 by one patient who had been rescued from kidney failure. 'I have cost the NHS tens of thousands of pounds—much more than I could have afforded privately; and although I am a member of BUPA it is a service that it does not provide because of the expense. Had my treatment depended on my ability to pay, I would not be alive today'. The speaker was Michael McNair-Wilson, who was then and is now Conservative MP for Newbury."

Robin Cook is the Shadow Secretary of State for Health & Social Security.

This pamphlet is based on a speech given at Guy's Hospital on 28 June 1988.

Cover design: Brian Nugent

August 1988

ISBN 0 7163 0529 1
ISSN 0307 7523

Printed by The College Hill Press Limited (TU), London & Worthing
Published by the Fabian Society, 11 Dartmouth Street, London SW1H 9BN

Life begins at 40: in defence of the NHS

On the fifth of July we celebrated the fortieth anniversay of the NHS. On the same date a Birmingham pensioner entered the Edgbaston Nuffield Hospital at the expense of *Retirement World*, a magazine aimed at the elderly, who sponsored a reader's hip operation as part of a commercial promotion. The company claimed apparently without any appreciation of the irony of the date, that this was Britain's first sponsored operation and as such it had been welcomed by Mrs Edwina Currie.

I have met too many pensioners waiting too long for hip replacements not to understand the relief she as an individual must have experienced that her waiting time was over. It was though wholly distasteful that her personal need for surgery should have been met as part of a marketing operation. And this new high in the commercial exploitation of health care provides only too accurate a pointer to the direction in which the NHS is being herded.

At forty the NHS is in danger of losing the attractive idealism of its youth and developing the world-weary, slightly cynical double standards of middle-age. Launching the Institute of Health Service Management (IHSM) submission to the Government Review last month Mr Ken Jarrold, a past president, observed that the NHS can no longer remain "an island of equality in an unequal society". That he added for good measure was "totally unrealistic". At the risk of getting even deeper into opprobrium with the IHSM, I would offer the general comment that there are still schools of political thought that query whether we should accept present inequalities as a fixed point of reference, and it is arguable whether some recent undoubted steps to wider inequality, notably the conjunction this spring of cuts in tax with cuts in benefit, really command consensus support within society. I believe that the equality of treatment on which the NHS was founded is not only better than the market in guaranteeing access to health care, it is also more efficient in allocating health resources.

Looking back over the debates of forty years ago it is interesting that no one then attempted to argue that the market had a role in allocating health care. True the Conservatives divided the Commons on both the Second Reading and the Third Reading of the National Health Service Bill, but on both occasions the focus of their opposition was a defence not of the market as the provider of health care but of charity as the source of hospitals for the poor. As their spokesman expressed it at the Third Reading, the charitable hospitals "are an outlet for private benevolence—and that is not a thing to be misprised". The debate was after all taking place against a background of health care which was in the main left to the market and no one could be found to defend the consequences.

Nor were those consequences solely that for the poor the reality of private health care was charity health care. It is striking that the bulk of the criticism of the previous situation in parliamentary debates did not concentrate on its inequity but on its stark inefficiency. Large tracts of the country had no real hospital provision and most operations were carried out by GPs doubling up as amateur surgeons. Julian Tudor Hart in his stimulating book to be published this autumn recalls joining such a practice in Kettering where a patient was once left under anaesthetic while a London specialist was summonded by the next train to rescue a stomach operation from which the local GP had retired baffled. Conversely in some large cities hospitals nestled in neighbouring streets, separately owned, separately managed and defiantly offering the same specialities in competition for the same paying patients (*A New Kind of Doctor*, Merlin Press).

It was Bevan's unqiue contribution not to compromise with this patchwork of ownership and control but to recognise that a single coherent structure of ownership and of funding was essential if he was to found a health service that offered universal access to a comprehensive range of treatment. The NHS has served us well in the intervening forty years. It provides a network of primary care that is largely without parallel in offering every citizen the right of access to a doctor within the community. It has developed a chain of district general hospitals that has brought specialised treatment to every significant population centre, whilst also sustaining centres of excellence that can rival any like hospitals around the world both in quality of training and innovation in research. It has removed anxiety over payment from the stress and pain of illness.

Moreover, it has achieved all this with great efficiency. Pride over the cheapness of the NHS can be misplaced as it partly reflects a long tradition of running the health service on poverty wages. However, it is the case that as a proportion of GNP, the National Health Service absorbs half as much as total expenditure on medical care in America whilst providing a demonstrably more comprehensive service. Giving evidence to the Select Committee, Dr Marvin Goldberg, Chief Executive of the American based AMI health group said the NHS provides: "Outstanding health care and British NHS hospitals are at least as good as those in America while British doctors are better".

A striking personal endorsement of the NHS was provided in 1984 by one patient who had been rescued from kidney failure, "I have cost the NHS tens of thousands of pounds—much more than I could have afforded privately; and although I am a member of BUPA it is a service that it does not provide because of the expense. Had my treatment depended on my ability to pay, I would not be alive today". The speaker was Michael McNair-Wilson, who was then and is now Conservative MP for Newbury.

In that passage he expressed much more accurately than his front-bench colleagues ever do the sense of security in the NHS which is one of the main reasons why it is so strongly valued by the public. And valued it still is. Despite all the adverse publicity last winter about the NHS on the brink of collapse, and despite the rash of propaganda

> **The NHS has served us well . . . It provides a network of primary care that is largely without parallel in offering every citizen the right of access to a doctor within the community. It has developed a chain of district general hospitals that has brought specialised treatment to every significant population centre . . . It has removed anxiety over payment from the stress and pain of illness. Moreover, it has achieved all this with great efficiency.**

plugging market medicine, the British public persists in giving the NHS their trust and their respect. This is partly because support for equity in health care is strongly rooted in popular culture, whatever tolerance there may be for inequality in other spheres. Recently, MORI discovered that the notion of a fast track within the NHS for those who paid extra was rejected by a majority of 2 to 1. Interestingly opposition to the proposal varied by only 2 per cent across social classes, indicating that its unpopularity is not simply a reflection of the shrewd assessment by the majority that they would be left in the slow track.

But popular support for the NHS is also based on the recognition of the greater efficiency of a planned public service over a market provision. The same MORI survey also found a 2 to 1 majority for the public sector in response to the question which sector would provide the better standard of health care if both had the same amount to spend.

The comparative efficiency of the NHS has also been endorsed by the regular external audits to which it has been subjected. The Guillebaud Report was commissioned by the Conservative Government of the fifties to identify how growth in health expenditure could be avoided, but disappointed its sponsors with its conclusion that "Any charge that there has been widespread extravagance in the National Health Service is not borne out by the evidence". Twenty-five years later, the Royal Commission on the NHS appointed by the Callaghan Government examined all the nostrums of alternative funding that have since been resurrected and rejected every one of them as less equitable in their outcome, more expensive to administer, and uncertain in any event to produce a significant increase in resources. They concluded, "In our review of the NHS as it exists we found much about which we can all be proud. Our examination of foreign health care systems for the most part reinforced that view".

The Government's Review

This popular support for the NHS and the habit of independent enquiries of producing clean bills of health for the NHS appears to have conditioned the character of the current Review. It is most unlikely to come up with conclusions that are politically inconvenient to the Government as it entirely consists of members of the Government—five of them, Mrs Thatcher, Nigel Lawson, John Major, John Moore and Tony Newton (now replaced by Kenneth Clarke). There are two immediate observations to be made about the structure.

First the block votes are weighted in the interests of the Treasury. The Prime Minister is herself technically a Treasury minister, but even if we assume, generously, that she is present as a dispassionate arbiter between Treasury and DHSS, it remains true that Nigel Lawson and John Major, who are both Cabinet ministers, outrank the DHSS representatives. The dominance of Treasury representation over DHSS representation mirrors the preoccupation of this administration with mechanisms of cost control rather than strategics of health care.

Secondly and more disturbingly is the limited character of the membership. It does not do justice to that limited character to describe it as a closed Review. It would be nearer the mark to describe it as hermetically sealed. There is no member of the Review team who has ever worked in the NHS. Indeed there was, until Kenneth Clarke's recent move, no member who was known to use the NHS. This is not Review by independent enquiry but Review by Cabinet sub-committee. Entertainingly in the first week after the Review was appointed the Table Office of the House of Commons declined to accept parliamentary questions about it, as internal Government committees officially do not exist.

Not that we have learnt much more since questions have been accepted. Ministers have refused to publish any of the evidence submitted to the Review as some of it *may* have been confidential. They have refused to name the organisations who submitted evidence on the imaginative grounds that "it would be impracticable to try to distinguish between those communications which see themselves as specifically 'submitting evidence' and those which do not, but which may, nevertheless, be relevant to the continuing review process".

Even our attempts to obtain the official remit of the Review have been baffled by the formula that the Review is "wide-ranging and fundamental".

Such a furtive Review may proceed swiftly and may reach ready agreement among its members. It is difficult to credit that meeting in private they will reach conclusions that will command sufficient public consensus to form the basis of a lasting reform.

Where a touch of franchising will result in a wider range of shops, cafes and hairdos for patients and staff I am all for it. I would not even oppose the NHS selling marketing and sponsorship opportunities within its hospitals, although it requires an effort to swallow my distaste at the ad-men invading this last refuge from their wiles and I hope we can at least spare nurses' uniforms from commercial sponsorship on the Adidas formula.

The role of the market

We do not as yet know what those conclusions may be. However, all the notes being dropped out of the window fit a consistent pattern of being concerned less with the quality of health care than with widening the role of the market in its provision—by increased competition, by more commercial medicine and by larger public subsidy of private medicine. In this respect the Review would appear to be on all fours with the trend of Government policy for the past decade, a period which has seen a consistent push to introduce the ethics of the market place into the health service.

Domestic and catering services have been made subject to competitive tendering. Only a fifth of contracts put out to competition have been won by private contractors in open tender and many of these have subsequently been surrendered when the company discovered it could not meet NHS standards of cleanliness and make a profit. However, the real significance of competitive tendering has been to impose private sector conditions of employment as the necessary basis on which in-house tenders can succeed. Domestic work is now increasingly performed by part-time casual staff with a high turnover who have seen wage rates decline as work norms have soared. An important element of the health team on the ward has been reduced with a corresponding increase in the workload of nursing staff. John Moore might not have been obliged to give such urgency to considering the case for introducing a new class of nurse assistants if he and his predecessor had not removed 70,000 domestics from the wards.

Existing charges for health care have been increased and new ones have been invented. Prescription charges are now 1,200 per cent higher than when the Government took office and exceeds the drugs cost of half of all prescriptions. For many common prescriptions it is now cheaper to pay the retail price and ministers presumably intend to foster a consumerist culture in which patients purchase their medication over the counter rather than have it prescribed through the health service. Dental charges are now set to recover three-quarters of the cost of treatment by an Act which gives ministers the power to increase the rate of recovered costs by order. It is entirely feasible that within the lifetime of this parliament the dental service will become self-financing, as has already happened with the optical service. The Government is accused of introducing charges for eyesight tests, but this does not do justice to the ideological character of their proposal. What the Government is proposing is the abolition of the fees they pay opticians for the service, leaving it to the market to determine the price which opticians will charge for this elementary preventive service.

There is a curious confusion about ministerial attitudes to charges. Although they are obliged by their economic doctrine to regard the price signal as effective in influencing demand in all other fields, in the case of health they are obliged to maintain that charges do not deter any patient from receiving treatment. Thus Tory Newton explicitly assured the Commons that, "There is no reason to expect people to be deterred from seeking eye tests". Markets seek equilibrium at the point where supply and demand are in balance. It would be a curious market which found equilibrium at the point at which no demand was unmet. By definition in leaving the price for tests to be struck in the market, ministers must expect some demand to be suppressed.

A third front for the commercial penetration of the NHS is supplied by the drive to increase private practice within the NHS. This it should be said has been a first-class commercial failure. In the lifetime of this Government the number of pay beds have been increased by a quarter, while over the same period the number of patients occupying them has fallen by a third.

This experience provides an instructive insight into the nature of retail competition in health care. NHS pay beds come backed by the guarantee of access to a range of technology and specialist expertise that few private hospitals can match. They are also cheaper than a bed in a private hospital, partly because health authorities are not at present supposed to run them at a profit. From the point of view of quality and of price, an NHS pay bed is the better buy. Unfortunately the private patients cashing in their BUPA policies expect to get for it the private bedroom with hotel furnishings as shown in the glossy brochure and know they will not get it at their district general hospital.

That is presumably why the IHSM submission to the Review requests the freedom to charge separately for higher standards of hotel charges. Personally I am entirely relaxed about patients being offered the option of going *á la carte* rather than *table d'hôte*, but it would be naive to imagine that this is primarily intended to widen choice for the NHS patient. Its primary purpose is to enable the NHS to compete more effectively for private patients.

This naturally brings me to the current enthusiasm for income generation. Where a touch of franchising will result in a wider range of shops, cafes and hairdos for patients and staff I am all for it. I would not even oppose the NHS selling marketing and sponsorship opportunities within its hospitals, although it requires an effort to swallow my distaste at the ad-men invading this last refuge from their wiles and I hope we can at least spare nurses' uniforms from commercial sponsorship on the Adidas formula. However, the problem with all these innovations is that the return for considerable diversion of managerial effort is very modest, and excessively modest if it is measured against the scale of NHS underfunding.

The dilemma of income generation is well expressed by Dr Ken Grant of City and Hackney, which is described in this field by the *Sun* as "pace-setting". Dr Grant has honestly observed that the real profits in income generation, not surprisingly, are to be found in "marketing what we are best at—our skills in the clinical field". It is clear that the Government sees income generation as leading to the marketing by the NHS of medical treatment and the current legislation is designed to remove the legal impediments to that goal. However, it is much less clear how an obligation to generate projects from the sale of health care can be reconciled with a duty to provide free access to comprehensive treatment.

It is important to set out fully the extent to which principles of the NHS have already been subverted by the deliberate encouragement of commercial pressures over the past decade, as this provides the background against which we must measure the outcome of the Review. Soothing murmurs are now being expressed to the specialist press correspondents that the Review will not go for revolution in the health service but will adopt a more evolutionary approach. The very fact that these reassuring noises are being made is a welcome admission that public support for the NHS remains too strongly entrenched for a frontal assault on it. Yet in practice all the Government appears to be promising is that it will carry on as before, taking a succession of Granny's footsteps, tiptoeing away from a universal, publicly-funded comprehensive health service hoping that no one will be sufficiently alarmed by the noise to ask the questions of principle raised by each step. It is a relief to know that the pace is not about to break into a stampede, but the time has come for the rest of us to ask the Government if the direction is right.

The right's remedies

I do not know precisely what the next step will be and am probably the last person in Britain whom the Prime Minister would choose to ring up at 1 am with an on-the-record statement. However, it is possible to identify the menu of choices before the Review by collating the submissions of their friends and former researchers who are now writing for the centres for ideological axe-grinding. The Adam Smith Institute, the Centre for Policy Studies and the Institute of Economic Affairs have so far this year extruded between themselves nine different tracts on making the health service more market controlled. This energy and fecundity which is certainly impressive should not be confused for width of intellectual support. Nearly all the authors come from a background as hired hands in political research, which is an honourable profession in its own way, but whose interests in the health service is secondary to their commitment to a set of ideological propositions. However, they do have the advantage over the rest of us that they have worked in Downing Street, and the even more marked advantage over the rest of us in being listened to in Downing Street. Let us therefore consider the remedies about which they are now telling Downing Street.

These may be grouped into three major headings:

- The funding of health care by insurance rather than taxation, to remove the explicit basis of health care as collectively rather than individually funded.
- Greater encouragement of private medical care, which often appears the main reason for advocacy of insurance funding which would put public and private contributions on the same basis and widen the scope for incentives to private health care through opt-outs.
- Greater competition within the public sector, and between the public and the private sector. There is a marked ambivalence about the latter element of competition, the same authors who advocate more open competition between public and private health care also call at different times for partnership between them. The problem for these authors is that their conviction that the public sector would benefit from competition is paralled by an anxiety to protect the private sector from all-out competition from the public sector. This is a perfectly normal political condition commonly known as wanting to have your cake and eat it.

it is simply not acceptable to most people that others should go in pain or risk premature death because they cannot pay the market price for treatment.

All these nostrums share the common feature that they are attempts to impose a market model on the provision of health care. There are though three limiting factors why health care cannot be reduced to a perfect market. First, with all respect to Mrs Currie, people do not choose to need medical treatment in the way that they choose to take a second holiday. The individual's requirement for health care over his or her life-cycle cannot be reasonably predicted by that individual and may well require expensive surgery or chronic treatment at a cost well beyond the resources of the individual.

Secondly, it is a rare individual who can correctly diagnose his or her condition and order the appropriate treatment for it from the local health retail outlet. Much more could be done by doctors, especially consultants, to counsel patients on alternative forms of treatment and to invite their participation in identifying the option with which they are most comfortable, but at the end of the day the consultant is paid to tell the patient what he or she thinks is wrong with the patient and what might put it right. The patient is not in the bargaining position of the consumer in any other situation of responding that he does not like that diagnosis and would like to buy another one.

Thirdly, there is the inconvenient feature of markets that they cater for demand rather than need, and satisfying the demand for health care at the market price may not be the same as meeting the social need for health treatment. In truth this is not a practical objection to a market in health care, but a political one. It is simply not acceptable to most people that others should go in pain or risk premature death because they cannot pay the market price for treatment.

The favoured model for promoting the market within the NHS is known as the internal market. Personally I can see merit in greater flexibility that permits health authorities to correct cross-boundary flows of patients with cross-boundary flows of cash. The National Association of Health Authorities has already identified three ways of achieving this, but I am content that we should experiment with a fourth method. However, there is no merit in the vision of the wider shores of the internal market in which competition would effectively become the basis of cash allocation within a public service.

Let us first clear away the undergrowth by removing a false prospectus. An internal market would not widen choice for the patients. Choice would be exercised by management who would decide which hospital offered the best buy. To that extent the scope for the patient, in consultation with the GP, to express a preference for a particular hospital would be reduced. Indeed implicit in the model of the internal market is the right of management to instruct patients that they will not be treated at the local District General Hospital because they have been placed in a bulk order at a better rate in another hospital.

The nub of the problem over the internal market is whether it is compatible with the objectives of the NHS to provide a full range of health service in each district. Can management become purchasing agents, concerned with striking the best bargain wherever it may be found and still be expected to take a comprehensive view of locally-provided services? Conversely, when they sell those services an internal market encourages them to put local needs secondary, as budgets are maximised by selling to the population of other districts.

The essence of competition is the expansion and contraction of competing firms. Are we really prepared to tolerate the logic of that approach with the NHS? Are we prepared, to sharpen the question, to accept health authorities shedding whole clinical specialities because they are an uneconomic line? And are we confident that the end result will not be regional monopolies and less patient choice?

Private insurance

The mechanism proposed to square the incompatibility of health care with the market is insurance. All market approaches to the NHS submitted to the Review stress the case for much wider private insurance and almost as frequently propose subsidies to boost it.

The first thing to be said is that private insurance does not offer to health care the alleged benefits of the discipline of the market place. At the point when the individual requires treatment he or she has already paid the premiums and has no incentive not to consume as expensive a treatment as can be reconciled with the policy. The position of the doctor is even more prejudiced in that he or she has every incentive to obtain as much as possible from the insurance company by recommending the most expensive treatment. Both patient and doctor are in a conspiracy to make the consultation as costly as possible, which is a perverse outcome for a proposal frequently floated by those who claim to be concerned about cost control.

The compulsion in an insurance-based system to maximise the rate of return is the simple explanation why intervention surgery is so much more often recommended in the United States. For example, the incidence of hysterectomy there is four times the British rate. This is unlikely to reflect higher morbidity rates but much more likely to reflect the greater willingness of doctors on a piece-work basis to recommend it, despite the operative risks and in the case of this particular operation the documented psychological trauma. I can guarantee that an expansion of private insurance will certainly meet the objective on increasing expenditure on health care, but it is not equally clear that the money will be spent effectively.

One direct diversion of resources imposed by any insurance-based scheme is the necessity for accountants and clerks and lawyers to assess costs and process claims. The NHS is routinely accused of excessive bureauracy, frequently I regret to say by the very people who work within it and are in a position to know it is not true. Expenditure on administration in the NHS is lower as a proportion of budget than the health system of any other nation, lower as a proportion of turnover than the private health sector within Britain, and come to that, lower than the management costs of just about any other major enterprise inside or outside the public sector. I am not myself sure that this is necessarily a feature of which we should be proud. On the contrary it is evidence of a persistent undermanaging of the NHS, which is largely responsible for its failure to exploit new developments in communication, cost control and personnel relations. Nevertheless, there is no more pointless expansion of administrative costs than the deadweight of those required to police and process an insurance-based system. These costs would be considerable.

Part of this additional cost burden is incurred in the task of hunting down bad debts, which does not contribute in any way to the provision of health care. Forty per cent of personal bankruptcies in the US are attributable to debts for medical care, a salutary reminder of the limitations set to insurance cover. These limitations have three dimensions.

First, insurance cover generally excludes those conditions which are chronic and therefore expensive, or complicated and therefore expensive. Standard exclusions in British insurance policies are arthritis, renal dialysis, multiple sclerosis or muscular dystrophy. Most people do not require substantial medical care until after retirement. Most insurance cover excludes the very

Expenditure on administration in the NHS is lower as a proportion of budget than the health system of any other nation, lower as a proportion of turnover than the private health sector within Britain and, come to that, lower than the management costs of just about any other major enterprise inside or outside the public sector.

conditions for which they are then most likely to require treatment. Short of retirement, the most expensive health care required by the majority of the population is maternity care, which is also excluded by the majority of insurance policies.

Secondly, insurance cover is generally restricted by upper limits which are arbitrary in every sense other than financial. I recently met a psychiatric consultant to a private clinic, who was prepared to discuss candidly the ethical dilemmas of treating patients whose financial cover is fixed at five weeks of residential care, but whose response to treatment may indicate that a longer period of hospitalisation is desirable.

Thirdly, insurance cover is further limited by exclusion of those most likely to claim on it. I am often struck at the sheer healthiness of the patients who illustrate the promotional literature of BUPA and PPP who appear in such pink of good cheer and fitness that it is difficult to figure out why they are in a hospital bed. These models are though in a sense most suitable for the purpose as the objective of insurance companies is to attract the healthy. They therefore claim the right to screen for the unhealthy and reject them from cover. This discriminatory approach was defended earlier this month by the managing director of WPA, Britain's third biggest health insurer, on the principled grounds that it meant "essentially healthy people are not penalised by unhealthy people". This statment has the advantage of originality in that it perceives healthy people as the vulnerable group and proposes a market remedy that protects them from the inconvenient costs of the unhealthy.

Given this limited character of health insurance in Britain, the private sector is patently not in a position to substitute for the NHS and to be fair most directors of BUPA or PPP would probably be horrified at the notion of accepting the comprehensive, open-ended liabilities of the NHS. It is therefore perplexing that so much effort in and around the Review appears to be addressed to the issue of how the private sector may be expanded rather than how the public sector may be improved. Two major devices are being canvassed to boost private cover—tax relief on private cover or opt-out from public cover, or for all I know both of them together. Both would be a major mistake.

Tax relief is open to the obvious objection that it targets help most on those who need it least—the healthy who are most likely to be accepted for private cover and the wealthy whose higher tax rates make relief most vulnerable. These are curious priorities for additional health expenditure.

Moreover, even in its own terms of stimulating higher spending on health, tax relief is likely to prove an ineffective mechanism. If for example the average premium is £200 pa the cost of tax relief for 6 million insured persons will be £300 million. The numbers under insurance need to increase by a third before the increased spending on premiums matches the cost of the subsidy and provides any net increase in health spending. Up to that point it will always produce a larger rise in health spending to increase the budget of the NHS by a sum equivalent to the cost of tax relief.

It is apparently being mooted that these objections could be circumvented by limiting the tax relief to the elderly.

At this point the proposal moves from the perverse to the eccentric. This restriction targets help for private insurance on the very group for whom private cover is most inappropriate as their most likely health needs are the ones most likely to be excluded from cover. Only a moment's reflection is required on the multiple ways in which we need to expand our health provision for the elderly to expose the hopeless irrelevance of tax relief as the solution for them.

Opt-out is even more objectionable. The basic problem with opt-out is that it requires the payment towards the NHS of every individual to be expressed in a manner that gives him or her something to opt-out from. The principal attraction to Leon Brittan of his proposal for an NHS insurance contribution appeared to be precisely that it paved the way for opting out (*A New Deal for Health Care*, Conservative Political Centre, 1988). Nor is this inconvenience confined to the need for a whole new element in the tax system. If one in ten of the population chose to opt-out, it would be the remaining nine out of ten who would have to prove they were not opted-out when they went along to seek treatment. With the new contributions comes a requirement to maintain a record of payment of them, and presumably a mechanism for credits to those not in work but who do not wish to be counted as having opted out of the NHS.

The more fundamental objection to both these proposals is that they explicitly threaten the NHS as a universal health service catering for everyone. Moreover, they threaten its universality in the worst possible way, by encouraging those with higher incomes and lower health needs to get out, leaving behind the less affluent and the less fit. In this respect such an approach to the NHS would be of a piece with the Government's strategy of erosion towards the rest of the social services—housing, pensions, and now education, where the Government has encouraged those who could afford it to opt-out of public provision, leaving behind the poor who could be expected to put up with a poor service.

Funding

This brings us to the real danger to the health service of a Government committed to expanding the private sector. The harsh truth is that the fastest way to drive people into going private is not to offer incentives that make the private sector more attractive, but to impose reduced standards that make the public sector less attractive. This is fully understood by the private insurance companies who make liberal use of NHS waiting lists in their promotional literature. A Government that chooses the rate of expansion of private medicine as the test of Government policy has a diminished commitment to removing the pressures on the NHS.

It was of course those pressures that prompted the Review in the first place. The Review was born out of a winter in which debate over the NHS was dominated by the underfunding of the hospital sector, made visible by closed wards and cancelled operations. The extent to which the Review was not premeditated but an urgent response to the political fallout of those events is neatly confirmed by its announcement only a fortnight after the Secretary of State has assured me that there was no Review of the NHS and there was no intention to appoint one. From the start those participating in the Review, whilst coy about its remit, have encouraged the view that the agenda is about identifying alternative funding for health care as the solution to its underfunding.

The problem now for the Review team is their difficulty in identifying alternative funding mechanisms that they can credibly present as resolving the original issue of underfunding—except possibly changing the law to permit larger lotteries. This leaves them with a major dilemma over how they navigate re-entry when their time is up. As a result I understand from journalists

The NHS is no longer presented as inherently flawed and ripe for fundamental reform. Apparently it is not really all that bad and just needs a bit of sprucing up. At this rate it will only be necessary to delay the Review a little further for the NHS to be rediscovered as a source of national pride.

that recently there has been a marked shift in the tone of background briefings. The NHS is no longer presented as inherently flawed and ripe for fundamental reform. Apparently it is not really all that bad and just needs a bit of sprucing up. At this rate it will only be necessary to delay the Review a little further for the NHS to be rediscovered as a source of national pride.

It is not so surprising in view of its origins that the Review has run into trouble. In the first place the design flaws in the funding mechanism most responsible for the crisis in underfunding was the tightening of cash limits in 1982 to exclude supplementary estimates for pay increases. As the standard textbook on NHS finance puts it, "In such circumstances one can only assume that this deliberate underfinancing of inflation was designed to engineer a cutback in service" (T Jones & M Prowle, *Health Service Finance*, Accountants Educational Trust, 1987). The recent decision to fund the nurses' pay settlement is a recognition that the previous practice has proved insupportable, but we can hardly expect the Review to make a formal admission of guilt.

The second and greater problem for the Review team is that in the absence of plausible methods of alternative funding, they have no cover left to conceal the unpalatable conclusion that the NHS is underfunded because it has been kept short of funds. A distinguished specialist journalist recently asked me if it was credible to claim that underfunding would be solved by more funding. With due temerity I would suggest that the claim is not only logical but, yes, credible.

In the first place even the most cursory skimming of comparative European spending levels suggests that Britain is trying to get its health service on the cheap. Curiously the New Right themselves frequently draw attention to this comparison in order to show that UK private health expenditure is lower than other European countries, but overlook that in absolute terms we are just as far behind in public expenditure on health, the remedy for which is much more in the Government's own hands.

It is striking how the international comparison has shifted adversely against Britain over the past two decades. From the founding of the NHS until 1960 public expenditure on health by Britain comfortably exceeded the OECD average expressed as a percentage of GNP. However, since then growth in health expenditure by other Governments has outstripped that of Britain. By 1970 Britain was only level-pegging with the OECD average and since 1980 we have been persistently below the OECD average, even although it is depressed by the low public health spending of the US. The inference is clear. The British problem is not essentially one of the mechanisms of funding, but of the shortage of funding. Indeed, it is even arguable that without the comparatively greater efficiency of the NHS our quality of health care would be even more conspicuously inferior to that of higher spending nations.

It also appears entirely credible to the overwhelming majority of the population that we both should and could make more funds available to the NHS. Immediately before the last Budget a remarkable 84 per cent of respondents stated that they would rather the Treasury surplus was put into the NHS than distributed in tax cuts. This is as near unanimity as we can hope to aspire to for almost any spending priority, and is a salutary reminder, confirmed by the subsequent Budget, that the political obstacle to higher health funding is not the reluctance of the public to pay for it, but the refusal of the Government to spend it.

Finally a higher level of health spending is also perfectly credible as a rational choice between competing economic priorities. Nothing has done more to maliciously undermine the case for an adequate NHS budget than the perverse conventions of the Treasury, which regards increased output of tobacco and alcohol as economic growth and therefore desirable, whilst increased provision for cancer and alcoholism is an inflation of public expenditure and therefore undesirable. As the Guillebaud Report expressed it: "It should not be forgotten, however, that the National Health Service is a wealth producing as well as a health producing service. In so far as it improves the health and efficiency of the working population, money spent on the NHS may be properly regarded as 'productive'—even in the narrow economic sense of the term".

Therefore, the notion of putting more funds into the NHS is neither eccentric nor profligate, but perfectly credible. Any outcome of the Government Review which claims to have resolved the pressures of underfunding without releasing additional funds will be wholly incredible. To those on the right who insist on describing greater investment in health care as throwing money at the problem, I would retort that at present there is nothing the NHS needs as much as having a bit of money thrown at it.

There is an alternative, and mildly more insulting, criticism of the advocacy of extra funds which is advanced from certain corners on the left. This turns on a simple and false dichotomy between new ideas and more funds. As a result those who advocate better funding of the NHS find themselves accused of being boring. It is a line of attack which draws on a long tradition of British intellectual elitism which has always harboured the suspicion that people who have money to spare are probably stupid.

New thinking

It is of course perfectly consistent to argue that the NHS needs both more funds and new ideas. The sterility of the Government's present approach is that it has confined the arena for new ideas to the narrow issues of alternative funding and managerial structure. The debate over the next forty years of the NHS ought to be a much wider and richer one about health care policy, not just accounting procedures. The studied disinterest which the Government has shown in those wider issues has created an unclaimed territory which the left can colonise—if that is not an offensive metaphor to apply to a leftist project. The results of Labour's own internal Review of health care will be published to coincide with the Government's review of alternative funding. Here are some of the questions on health care policy which we are currently examining.

First, how do we measure cost effectiveness in health care. We are surprisingly ignorant as to whether what we actually do in hospitals is the best way of promoting health care. We also show an astounding indifference as to whether it is successful. The Government is now requiring hospitals to supply several hundred entries of data as part of the Korner measures of performance. All of them measure performance in terms of quantity of throughput rather than quality of outcome.

We need measures of quality control, not just productivity from our health service.

There is also the separate question of whether patients are treated not just with competence but with respect. We need a patients' charter that provides a checklist against which they can measure any hospital. Did it provide an individual appointment time? Was it

Any outcome of the Government Review which claims to have resolved the pressures of underfunding without releasing additional funds will be wholly incredible. To those on the right who insist on describing greater investment in health care as throwing money at the problem, I would retort that at present there is nothing the NHS needs as much as having a bit of money thrown at it.

kept to? Was the reception welcome and reassuring? Were there childcare facilities? Did the consultant or junior explain their diagnosis and discuss alternative forms of treatment? How flexible were the visiting hours? In the Second Reading debate forty years ago Bevan observed that he would rather recover in the sterile efficiency of a large hospital than expire in a warm gush of sympathy in a small one. But is there any reason why we cannot devise methods of personalisation that give us general hospitals with both efficiency and warmth?

Associated with responsiveness to the patient is accountability to the local community. I recently discussed a closure decision with a management that could tell the proximity of the replacement facility to the nearest tenth of a mile, but could not tell me the number of changes of bus required to get there. It was an interesting insight into the manner in which decisions are taken by people who never use public transport affecting consumers, particularly the elderly, disabled and mothers of young children, who are dependent on public transport. Health authorities need to become more representative of the people they serve and less representative of ministers.

They should also be formed in a way that obliges them to take a wider view of health needs in their community. As someone familiar with the integrated health boards of Scotland, I remain perplexed why in England anyone imagines that it makes sense to manage primary care through a different authority from the management of hospitals, or even more curiously from the management of community services. As a result family planning clinics are being closed around England because it has the happy effect of passing the cost of the service on to someone else's budget. The simplest solution to the problem of out of hours cover within the inner cities would be a deputising service as an extension of the accident and emergency units who receive those without adequate cover in any event, but such a solution is made unthinkable by the institutional separation of the two health agencies.

Integration would also assist in evolving the health service from a reactive service treating disease, to a proactive service promoting health. Edwina Currie has single-handedly almost succeeded in giving preventive health a bad name by seeking to capture it for the individualist ideology of the New Right. However, any serious programme of health promotion must be addressed to issues that go much wider than individualist lifestyles and require collective action from the Government. The mass adoption of a healthy diet is not possible without a national food policy that restores nutritional standards to schools and obliges the food processing industry to justify and disclose the non-nutritional content of its products. Promotion of exercise requires a willingness to invest in leisure facilities, or at any rate keep open the ones we have got. Only government and not the individual, certainly not the consumer, can ensure that the real cost of tobacco and alcohol is increased, although that could produce a greater gain in health outputs than any other single measure.

Related to health promotion is the challenging data on inequalities of health. These are persistently ignored by those who perceive health promotion as solely a matter of individual lifestyles, but the consistency with which low income families achieve higher morbidity rates and lower indices of health such as child growth, cannot be explained away as the invariable choice of inferior lifestyles by the individuals making up this class. In large part the inequalities in health across society mirror inequalities in income and the evidence of the past decade is that both have widened in parallel with each other. No programme is likely to reduce health inequalities unless it reverses the recent measures that increase poverty in our society, but at the same time health agencies must ask why those who have the highest need for health care appear the least effective in demanding it.

They are unlikely to find the answers if their role is confined to responding to the individual aspirations of patients as consumers without taking a view of the overall needs of the community they serve. Fortunately here the necessary questions have already been asked and answered in the Acheson Report on Public Health. What is now needed is action to implement its recommendations that health authorities are given an explicit duty to monitor the health of the public in their area and review annually progress towards specific objectives for its improvement.

It would also be sensible to set annual targets for progress in community care. Press focus on acute cases turned away from the surgical wards, tends to obscure the even more seriour underfunding of the chronic sector. It is one of the paradoxes that the mentally handicapped or psychiatrically ill who stay longest in hospital, frequently are expected to do so in the oldest and most dilapidated buildings with the poorest staffing ratios. How do we provide for them alternative less institutionalised care in the community? Whilst we might welcome the lead role of local authorities outlined by Griffiths, do we accept the limitation that Griffiths imposed on that role by defining local authorities as the purchasers of residential places not as their provider? We need to provoke the vigorous debate on Griffiths which the Government evaded by slipping out the report without public statement while the author was under the anaesthetic.

Finally, any examination of the NHS can only be complete if it takes full account of its responsibilities within the labour market, where it is Britain's largest employer. How do we balance our desire to improve services to the patient with our duty to provide a fair reward to staff? Not only are NHS wage rates themselves a major source of poverty in work, but inequalities within the NHS have widened as a result of the growing gap between staff covered by the Pay Review Body and those staff outwith it. How do we achieve improvements in nurse staffing against a background of declining numbers in the age group from which they are recruited? That demographic challenge may even be beneficial if it obliges us to find a strategy for nurse staffing that differs from Haig's policy at the Somme of burning up successive intakes of eighteen year olds.

Regrettably, these do not appear to be questions being asked by the ministers on the Review team. These are, nevertheless, the issues we should be addressing if we want to see the NHS shake off its mid-life crisis and face the next forty years with confidence. If we resolve them successfully there is every reason to believe that the NHS could prove that it really is true that life begins at forty.